the Diet

the Diet

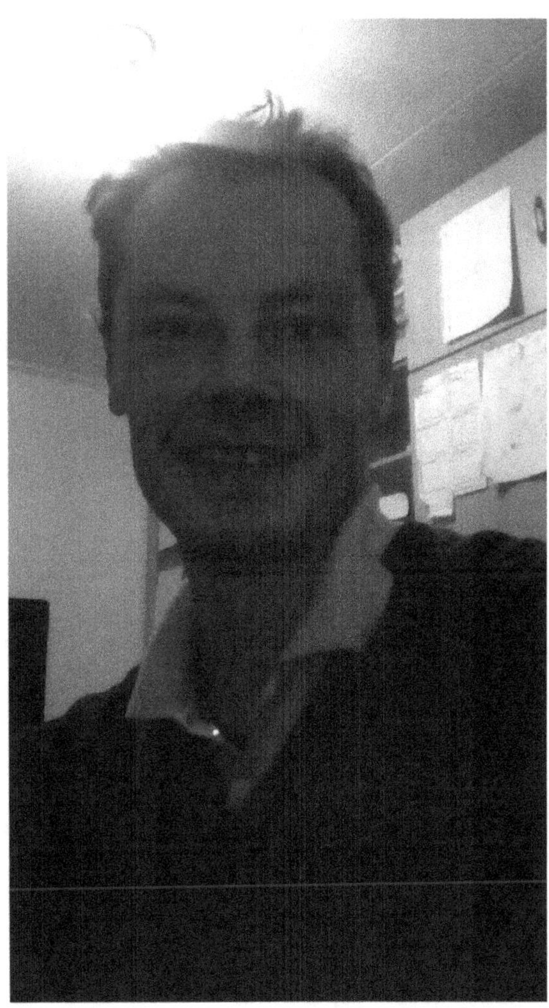

Jasmin Hajro

Jasmin Hajro

© 2020 Jasmin Hajro

Written by Jasmin Hajro

Selfpublished by Jasmin Hajro

Cover design by

Jasmin Hajro

First edition 2021

<u>Victory….</u>

<u>The bio of author Jasmin Hajro, nice to meet you</u>

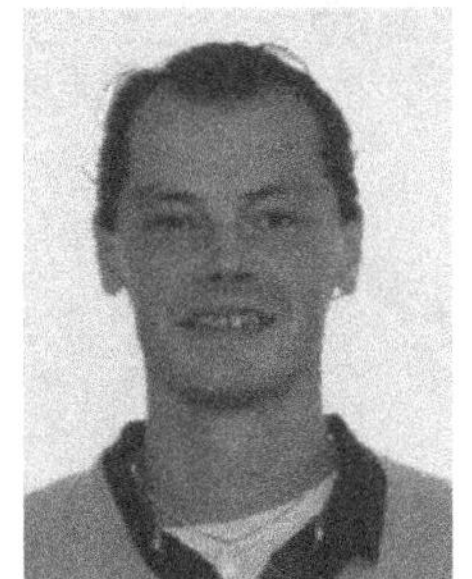

Hello dear reader, how are you ?
Thank you for buying my book Victory

.

My name is Jasmin Hajro,
I was born on July 6, 1985 in Bosnia.
As refugees, we came to the Netherlands 21 years ago.
After having completed school & worked at several jobs ...

On 17 December 2012, I founded my first company: investment firm Jasko.
After a successful first year, I unfortunately had to close that company. After a short period of rest, unemployment and temporary work. I started again as an entrepreneur.

On September 1, 2015, I founded establishment Hajro.

(We say establishment instead of company,
because we do a bit more then just sell stuff.
Like providing jobs,
donating to 40 different charities,
and helping people to live richer.)

Since the beginning the core activity is,
selling sets of greeting cards, door to door.
Nowadays the product range has been expanded.

With, among other things, the selling of my 10 books.

The royalties of my books are donated to the charity: foundation Giveth Life.

My company is now part of Hajro Group,
which consists of 20 different subsidiaries,

that are part of 1 umbrella organization :
Called Energy Now.

For more information about my company
& the foundation,
go to my website : **www.hajro-international.webnode.nl**

You can find my books at my author website :
www.jasminhajro6.webnode.nl

Victory

Hello again...

I am Jasmin Hajro,
and you just have read a few things about me
in my bio.

But you have bought this book because you
want to know the whole story.

My life story ....

I called it Victory,
because I have overcome a few things.

I am 32 years old and live in Doetinchem,
in the Netherlands.
I work as a salesman
on behalf of Hajro.
I sell sets of greeting cards,
gift mugs and booklets.

Part of the proceeds go to more than 15 Charities.

You can find everything about establishment Hajro at
www.hajro.be (dutch website)

I now live in the Netherlands.

But on 6 July 1985 I was born in Sarajevo,
in Bosnia.

When I was a young child, we lived in Gora.
That is a village in Bosnia.
It is on a mountain.
A mountain village.

The view is great,
lots of nature.
Clean, fresh air.

I remember it as a happy time.

The house we lived in
was a kind of 2 houses under 1 roof.
Aunt Rahima had lived in the other part.
Until her own house was built.

My parents both worked,
and I went to Biba,

an elderly woman in the village,

that was my babysitter.

I remember she had an old-fashioned stove,

which worked on firewood.

And we placed unripe walnuts

behind the stove, to ripe.

Under our house,

you had a steep part of soil,

and below that a flat piece of land.

On that flat piece of land,

we grew vegetables,

potatoes and very small tomatoes.

There were also pear trees and walnut trees growing there.

My mother worked at Tas,

an automobile factory,

where they made or processed.

small car parts.

I do not remember anymore

what kind of work my father did then ...

You notice that it has been a very long time ago.

I was always very happy to see him,

when he came home.

And asked once if he could work 2 days a week,

and be free 5 days a week.

My uncle Ibro lived close to us,

with Aunt Sevda and my nieces :

Sanela and Amela.

They had a red swing.

I have been swinging on it and went

as high as possible,

Until I got a kind of butterflies in my stomach feeling,

by excitement.

I do not know how to exactly describe that feeling.

With my cousins I did play games such as hide & seek.

I once wrestled with my father

and then I ended up falling weird on my wrist,

it hurted.

Then Dad said: hajmo kod Ibre rostiljat

Let's go barbequing at Uncle Ibro.

I went to the mosque,

and learned prayers

and how to pray.

I asked the hodza

that's a kind of reverend,

how you can know if someone is lying.

He said you can see it on the forehead.

That it turns a little red.

It is very peaceful in the mosque,

I still see it that way.

Although it has been a while since I visited one.

————————

It is now March 27, 2018,

00:44 hours at night.

I'm getting out of bed in the mornings, late again....

I wake up at 9 or 10 in the morning

from the alarm clock.

I then switch off the alarm.

And fall asleep again.

When I wake up again afterwards it is already noon.

I had sleeping pills a few weeks ago,

for 2 weeks..

It went well

I started going to bed earlier,

and getting up earlier. Before noon.

Maybe it is a strange time, in the middle of the night

to write a book.

But I thought that once, I just had to start writing it.

When I was playing at Chess Club Doetinchem,

I said to Frans that I wanted to write a book

about my life.

That could have been in 2009.

————————————

Biba, the woman who looked after me when my parents worked,

was also the babysitter of an orphan.

I do not remember what his name was.

But we went to the mosque together.

There he farted ...

And we were both thrown out.

My father drove a Fico,

that is like a kind of old model Fiat 500 car.

If we drove to Grandpa and Grandma,

I could sit on Dad lap

behind the wheel.

The first time I saw snow,

I walked outside in my pajamas.

I was completely stunned to look at it.

Amazing.

It must have been cold outside.

The winters in Bosnia are colder than here.

My father became very angry,

and I got a beating with his belt.

I remember that I was rolling over the ground

and called: nemoj babo

Don't hit me, Dad

My index finger was completely swollen,

because I was hit there too.

I still love it

to look outside

when it snows.

Everything seems so peaceful then.

Oh, those beatings were normal.

That was how you got punishment,

and how other children received punishment

in Bosnia.

I was 6 years old when I went to school for the first time.

When my sister, Emina was born and I saw her for the first time, she looked tinted. And I thought
she was not my sister.

My father once had in an angry mood,

thrown the TV out of the window.

I have around my twentieth year

done the same thing once.

Once my father went to Aunt Rahima,

and I was not allowed to go with him.

Then I went outside

and looked in through the window at them.

My father got angry,

and I had to sit naked in front of the house.

If I wanted a beating,

then I could ask

my daddy, he told me.

My father drank,

mom says he beat her too.

The war had started

between Bosnia and Serbia.

We had moved

because the enemies came too close.

We have moved a number of times.

My father had to fight for Bosnia,

in the battlefield. And was not always with us.

We left the village

and we were in an abandoned house.

I do not remember what that place is called.

We have harvested grain,

and grown potatoes.

We took care of the cow of uncle Ibro,

Galava.

On my fathers request, I had tied Galava to a tree,

so she could graze grass.

But I hadn't shortened the chain

and she had too much

walking space

so she had eaten a number of our potato plants.

I got another beating.

You could hear the shooting from a distance.

A house near the one where we were in, was blown up.

We left that place in the evening.

A previous hotel became at that time

a shelter for refugees.

We spent a while there,

and got food packages.

I also fell on the stairs there

with a bottle of milk,

and had a cut on my wrist.

It is been stitched and the scar

looks like a cross.

You can still see it,

on my left hand.

My father was not with us

in that shelter.

I remember that we were waiting one time,

with lots of people,

probably for those foodpackets.

It was so oppressive ...I felt like I was choking.

My aunt Rahima had already fled to the Netherlands,

and they arranged that we could go there too.

I remember that I had to hold my sister's hand

and was not allowed to let go. When we were with the cow

walking through the forest.

I do not know how long we have walked.

My father stayed behind at a border.

And said to mom

prepare today for tomorrow &

prepare tomorrow for the day after tomorrow

We had help from a woman in Croatie.

Eventually we were awaited somewhere

by Aunt Rahima.

We signed in as refugees.

And went to an asylum seekers center,

a period of time in Alkmaar ..

And a period of time in Kampen near Dronten.

There, I watched Lion King for the first time and

almost had to cry,

because I missed my father.

We went to school and learned Dutch.

After the asylum seekers' centers we got a Roahuis

in Doetinchem,

on the Leliestraat. (lilystreet)

(a Roa house meant that we had a house and

the government paid the costs for living,

if I remember correctly)

After 5 years we received the Dutch nationality.

It was a red appartmentbuilding on the Leliestraat,

where we lived.

We got to know Zihra,

who lived in the blue building.

Also from Yugoslavia.

There were 3 brothers in our red flat,

a few houses further.

One of them had hanged himself.

My father came to the Netherlands wounded.

We had those piggy banks,

in which we saved money.

So that dad could come to us.

It would be like before,

our family together .....

I played a fighting game with Dad on the Nintendo.

And he made baked eggs in the morning.

Very tasty.

The reunification did not last long.

My father left us.

My parents then divorced.

We got a rental house in Doetinchem,

at the Ottawastreet 19.

We are still living there now.

Although mom now has a boyfriend,

and is with him in the weekends.

And my sister Emina,

is now very pregnant.

I will be an uncle,

in a few weeks.

I once already had described on paper

this piece of my life :

my time in Bosnia and

the flight to the Netherlands.

And called it Rebel.

With more details,

but I lost it.

Or someone took it.

After group 8 I went to the MAVO.

At the Rietveld lyceum in Doetinchem.

I obtained the Mavo diploma.

The Mavo lasts 4 years,

I think in the 3rd year

of the Mavo,

I had moved and lived with my father for a while.

In Smilde, province of Drenthe.

Then I came back to mom.

Heartbroken.

____

I think this will become a series ......

Are you looking forward to the sequel?

To be continued.

Thank you for reading

the first part of my life story.

<u>Victory II</u>

<u>The bio of author Jasmin Hajro, nice to meet you</u>

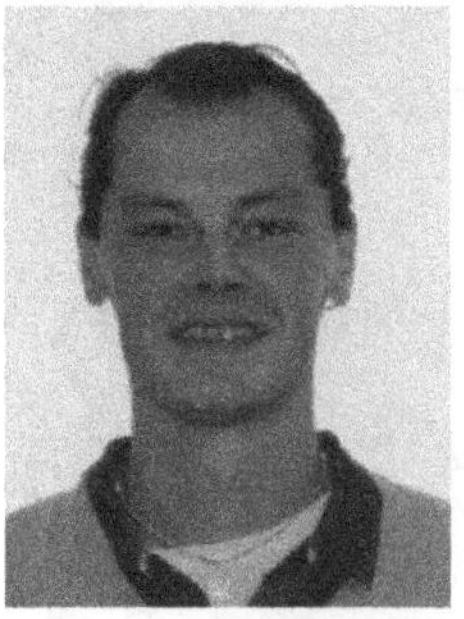

Hello dear reader, how are you ?

Thank you for buying one of my books.

My name is Jasmin Hajro,
I was born on July 6, 1985 in Bosnia.
As refugees, we came to the Netherlands 21 years ago.
After having completed school & worked at several jobs ...

On 17 December 2012, I founded my first company:
investment firm Jasko. After a successful first year,
I unfortunately had to close that company.

After a short period of rest, unemployment and temporary work.
I started again as an entrepreneur.

On September 1, 2015, I founded establishment Hajro.

(We say establishment instead of company,
because we do a bit more then just sell stuff.
Like providing jobs,
donating to 40 different charities,
and helping people to live richer.)

Since the beginning the core activity is,
selling sets of greeting cards,
door to door.
Nowadays the product range has been expanded.

With, among other things, the selling of my 12 books.

The royalties of my books are donated to the charity:
foundation Giveth Life.
From there more than 40 other charities
receive donations.
And by buying this book, so do you.
Thank you.

My company is now part of Hajro Group,
which consists of 19 different subsidiaries,
that are part of 1 umbrella organization.
Called Energy Now (Energie Nu)

For more information about my company
& the foundation, go to www.hajrobv.nl

<u>prelude book Victory III</u>

Hello Friend,
how are you ?

Is it weird that I call you friend?
If you have bought and read Victory & Victory II,
and you also bought Victory III,
to read.
Then you put so much trust in me,
like a friend does.

Thank you for being a loyal reader,
I really appreciate it.

I said that the proceeds (royalties)
from my books go to the Giveth Life foundation,
and that from there more than 40 other Charities
receive donations.

So, by buying this book,
you now also support,
more than 40 good causes.

Thank you & congratulations.

I should not actually do this ...
But you have shown so much faith in me.

It would be good then,
to prove to you,
that what I say,
also really happens.

So I trust you,
that you deal confidentially with it,
with that proof.
Ok?

SNS — 44 2018, blad 2/6

Zakenrekening
NL09 SNSB 0705 9732 71

Datum		Bedrag	Omschrijving
19-06	AF	0,25	PERIODIEKE OVERBOEKING NAAR NL73 INGB 0003 3377 37 stichting diva dichtbij Gift, hajrobv.nl
19-06	AF	0,25	PERIODIEKE OVERBOEKING NAAR NL54 RABO 0110 4360 08 voedselbank doetinchem Gift, hajrobv.nl
19-06	AF	0,25	PERIODIEKE OVERBOEKING NAAR NL68 RABO 0132 2355 36 Koninklijke nederlandse politiehondenvereniging Gift, hajrobv.nl
19-06	AF	0,25	PERIODIEKE OVERBOEKING NAAR NL49 RABO 0133 9780 95 stichting Joni Gift, hajrobv.nl
19-06	AF	0,25	PERIODIEKE OVERBOEKING NAAR NL25 RABO 0231 9575 48 VIOD Gift, hajrobv.nl
19-06	AF	0,25	PERIODIEKE OVERBOEKING NAAR NL14 ABNA 0533 4404 59 penningmeester S.V. doetinchem Gift, hajrobv.nl
19-06	Bij	36,82	DE66 3006 0010 9999 9390 28 COTR0289089/4-DE66300600010999993 9028-KOBO INC PUBLISHER PAYMENTS (Acc.: K01224)-ROYALTY PAYMENT WL00042062
20-06	AF	0,25	PERIODIEKE OVERBOEKING NAAR NL47 RABO 0312 3985 73 stichting vrienden van het Slingeland ziekenhuis Gift, hajrobv.nl
20-06	AF	0,25	PERIODIEKE OVERBOEKING NAAR NL23 RABO 0333 7779 99 kwf kankerbestrijding Gift, hajrobv.nl
20-06	AF	0,25	PERIODIEKE OVERBOEKING NAAR NL24 ABNA 0428 9798 15 stichting sportclub only friends Gift, hajrobv.nl
20-06	AF	5,00	PERIODIEKE OVERBOEKING NAAR NL42 RBRB 0919 2626 51 stichting laat het zieke kind genieten Gift, hajrobv.nl
20-06	AF	11,25	NL20 SNSB 8815 8669 14 STICHTING GIVETH LIFE
20-06	AF	18,41	NL20 SNSB 8815 8669 14 STICHTING GIVETH LIFE

You've seen a bank statement,
from the account number of the
Giveth Life Foundation.
You see that my book revenue
(royalties)

have been paid out, by Kobo.

And you see evidence,
that every day donations are made to
Charities,
with modest amounts.
And monthly with a larger amount.

(stichting means foundation)

The donations,
that goes on every day & every month ...

I set that up,
that it goes automatically.

Because I am the founder & treasurer
from the Giveth Life foundation.

And you are now a donor &
support more than 40 Charities,
because you bought this book.

Wooohoooo

Together with you we support :

Foundation Let the sick child enjoy, Mini manna foundation, Doctors without borders, Kika
(children with cancer), West Achterhoek Library,Natural monuments 's Graveland Association,
Save the children, AAP foundation, Cliniclowns,
Achterhoek Animal Center, VIOD, Gasthuisfonds, Animalfate Foundation, Royal Dutch police dog
association, Joni Foundation, Chess Association Doetinchem, NDD Swimming Association,
Kidney Foundation,
foundation Energy 4 all, Cordaid, foundation friends of the Slingeland hospital, foundation diva
nearby, Kwf cancer control, foundation mama cash, Warchild, Chance fund, Lepra foundation,
Refugeeswork Netherlands,
Food bank Doetinchem, Doetinchem hockey club, Free press unlimited, Orange Fund, Animal
Protection, Mother Teresa Foundation National MS fund, Noordbikers, Plan Nederland, Heart
foundation, Scouting Netherlands Fund, Unicef, Light for the World, Terre des Hommes
Foundation,

Humanitas Association, Greenpeace Foundation, Cheer up Foundation, Children's Stamp
Foundation, Tuberculosis Foundation, Baby Hope Foundation,UAF Foundation, Alzheimer's
Foundation, Parkinson's fund, Thomas relief fund Madras, World Wildlife Fund,
Homeless people foundation, Rudolph foundation, V.V. Doetinchem, foundation Youth Sports
Fund,
Amnesty International, Bartimeus Sonneheerdt association &
Handicapped sports in the Netherlands.

This is how we contribute together,
to a better world.

Together we can give more.

Now you also understand why you can buy
a paid version of
book Recipe for Happiness.
While you can also get the free version.
Because the book is the same.

You can give the paid version as a gift,
while you also support more
than 40 Charities.

That way you get a feeling of fullfillment,
by purchasing the paid version.

End of prelude.

<u>book Victory II</u>

Hi dear reader,

how are you ?

I am Jasmin Hajro,

and you just have read a few things in my bio

about me.

But you have bought this book because you

want to know the whole story.

My life story ....

I called it Victory,

because I have overcome a few things.

So, I am Victorious. And you as a donor of more than 40

charities are Victorious too.

Did you enjoy Victory ?

Sorry for the spelling mistake in it.

Welcome to Victory II

I am 32 years old and live in Doetinchem,

in the Netherlands. I work as a salesman

on behalf of Hajro.

I sell sets of greeting cards,

gift mugs and booklets.

Part of the proceeds go to Charities.

You can find everything about it at

www.hajrobv.nl

It's now March 31, 2018,

23:52 hours.

On this Saturday I am free ....

Well,

I have prepared the presents for customers today,

and also the business cards and mugs. For next week.

I bought some groceries,

vacuumed the house. And have eaten 3 times.

Then I went for a run.

It was half past 10 in the evening.

It also started to rain

and I was soaking wet after my jogging lap.

Then I smoked some tabacco and

drank a cup of tea.

But do not tell anyone.

Yes, I smoke tabacco,

and I jog.

There are no excuses for not exercising.

If a smoker can do it,

then you can certainly do it too.

After showering,

I ate my midnight snack.

A piece or 6 sandwiches with cheese

and a glass of milk.

My sister and her husband have returned

from a wedding and have went

to bed.

Beamy our cat, also came home.

Maybe you think that I've written and published ,

a lot of books in a short period of time ....

That is not a mystery.

First of all, my books are short.

I believe you do not need to write an encyclopaedia,

to teach someone something.

We used to have an offer at the Hajro E-store,

the VIP. That is a luxury greeting card subscription,

where you get all kinds of extra bonuses.

The Recipe for Happiness would be included for free.

And it would be about one page long.

But it is now a comprehensive

valuable guide,

and become a nice book.

You know the period when there were so many people

fired at the banks ...

I then got a good idea

By means of a program,

the bank could help people to become rich

and instead of firing employees, keep them and

hire new staff.

Tired and feverish, I had neatly typed out my program.

And I went to ING bank with it.

They did not want it.

And that program became my book

the lifebuoy for banks " loyal banking "

As you can see, the book was basically ready.

I have many years ago

written a number of poems .

It has also been years since I had been sending messages

and jokes via Facebook

to Rietje. (A girl I fell in love with, who had been a coworker)

I had printed out all those messages

and put them in a folder.

So my book Poems, jokes and book,

was also largely finished.

If I ask you to describe me

how your day was today ...

That would not be that difficult for you.

If I asked you to describe how your

past month was.

Then that too, would not be difficult for you.

So for my book Victory,

it was a matter of sitting down

rolling up my sleeves and starting to write.

I just described how

my life has been in that period of time.

So, therefore,

Well, you now know how I , in short chunk of time,

have been able to write & publish a number of books.

Ok, that being said, where were we ?

When I did the MAVO education

(general secondary education If I translate correctly),

I had lived with my father for a while.

And returned heartbroken to mommy.

It had hurt me a lot,

when my father left us. When we lived in Lilystreet

(Leliestraat)We had missed him for so long,

and had those piggy banks

in which we saved money,

so that dad could come to us. From Bosnia.

And after being reunited for such a short time,

he left us.

Maybe then as a child I thought,

that he did not want us,

and that he did not want me.

So he went to live in Smilde,

we stayed in Doetinchem.

I missed him very much,

and wanted to live with him.

My mother had a boyfriend at the time

who then drove me to dad, I believe.

My father had a new wife,

she is Dutch,

and has 2 daughters from her previous marriage.

I went to the Nassau college there,

in Assen. I had to every morning

travel for 1 hour on my bicycle to get to school.

I especially liked going to my aunt

Kasema , and spending time with my cousins.

Aunt Kasema is Papa's younger sister.

She has 2 sons and 1 daughter.

We played super mario

on a game computer.

And had lots of fun.

At school things were going ok.

I could hardly share my father at home

with them.

In principle, we were nice to each other.

I started my puberty then, I think.

I was pulled back and quiet.
I listened to rap music.

At school I was friends with Robert,
who called himself Skip.
In the break we were once driving around
on his scooter. I was on the back seat.
A bit driving through the city,
and in front of the police station,
without helmets on.

Then we slipped and fell down while taking a curve.

My father was not happy.

This is how the tensions built up at home ..
In the end I could choose
either change my behavior or return to my mother.

So I went back to mom, sad.

I went through the 4th class of the Mavo
at the Ludger college.

I then started to smoke.

Cigarettes. To try what it was like.

The first time I became dizzy.

Then it became a habit.

Then I started to smoke weed.

To try it.

I never liked the smell.

It was funny at first, with periods of time in which I started

laughing at almost anything.

Then that became a habit.

And it seemed like I was less active.

I had been practising karate for more than a year.

I was stoned every weekend.

Watching movies, eating chips.

Hanging around.

I became friends with Kai,

a classmate.

We had fun.

We got one time

a block of hash,

to sell.

We eventually ended up smoking the whole thing ourselves.

We have that movie, Pulp Fiction

seen about 20 times.

Very very stoned.

Just so often,

that we had memorized the dialogues from the film.

Like :

Ezekiel 25:17

the path of the rightious man

is beset on all sides

by the enequeties of the selfish

and the tyrrany of evil men

Blessed is he

who in the name of charity

and goodwill

Shepperds the weak

through the valley of darkness

And I will strike down upon thee

with great vengeance

and furious anger

Those who attempt to poison and destroy my brothers

And you will know

that my name is the lord

When I lay may vengeance

upon thee....

I even now remember the lines.

Ridiculous right ?

Maybe we have seen that movie 30 times.

Later I started to experiment with other drugs.

Xtc tablets and speed.

Of course I had tasted my very first beer,

a while ago.

So I often drank beer and smoked weed

to become strunk.

Stoned and drunk. At the same time.

I went way over my limits,

and had to vomit quite some times

because of too much booze.

I started to go higher more often

with those pills.

When taking them, you feel really good,

you gett energy from them,

and I went to drink a lot of coffee

so that the effect lasted longer.

Eventually I was awake all night after taking 5 pills,

and just continued to take even more.

We sat in a park with some people who I

did not know.

Me and Pino. That's what everyone called him.

I also sniffed some speed and drank red vodka.

At a given moment,

we started walking home.

And was it was like I could see the wind.

I had taken 10 or 15 tablets.

I began to hyperventilate.

When we arrived at home it was already morning ...

I was looking very pale,

and wanted to drink water but couldn't.

I walked back and forth,

could not stop.

I thought my chest would explode.

In a hallucination, I saw a big black hole,

thought I was going to die

and peed in my pants.

My mother and sister had come down

and panicked.

I think someone called the police

and I was thrown into a van.

Then the lights went out,

I lost consciousness.

I woke up in a hospital bed.

My father came and asked if I knew what I looked like.

I said no.

My face was swollen.

I had been in a coma for several hours.

They had said to my mother:

if he does not wake up,

then he will not survive.

This happened in a point of time in my life ,when I was

working in the hospitality industry , at restaurant the Mirror (de Spiegel).

Pretty quickly after my neardeath experience,

I went back to work again.

I came to work a few times too late

and was fired there.

I have tried the Havo education,

(higher general secondary education)

the adult education program,

but that did not work out.

I registered at temporary employment agencies

and worked at jobs that they offered me.

Mainly productionwork.

I have after that coma,

once tried to smoke a joint.

I didn't feel good,

got palpitations.

That was the last time.

From then on, I stopped taking drugs.

I did still drink alcohol.

And now also whiskey.

It often went with those jobs

the same way..

I did it for a while.

I worked, earned.

Started to show up late.

And was fired

or

did not show up anymore.

I applied for a job in 2007

at Palestra / Landal,

and started working as a dishwasher.

I came too late there, too

though I did not have to start working until the afternoon.

There was a positive atmosphere,

and we always had a drink after work with coworkers.

Once I got at home, I kept on drinking.

I was allowed to help on the cold side of the kitchen,

to prepare appetizers and desserts.

After some time, I was fulltime on the cold side.

Eventually I also learned the warm side of the kitchen,

making soups. Baking fish and steak.

Cooking lunch and dinner.

I worked hard,

I wanted to live better.

One day after my birthday,

after I had drunk a lot.

I collapsed and fell to the floor.

(Perhaps becaue of too much drinking and fatigue)

I then stopped drinking alcohol.

I had a permanent job there.

The work became hard to do,

until I didn't funtion there at all anymore.

I got resigned.

Then I was at home and had the feeling

that I broke down.

I received a unemployment benefit.

In the last years that I had worked there,

I started watching motivating

videos on yooutube.

From Jim Rohn and Brian Tracy.

I also received a journal as a gift, an empty book to write in.

While working at Landal,

I earned well and had few expenses.

I saved and did a homestudy course :

Wiser with money.

Then I learned to invest myself.

By taking another homestudy course,

read books about investing

and by investing myself.

Somewhere I read about pensions

and the pension discount.

If you have worked abroad for a number of years

or are a immigrant and have not 67 years of employment history,

then you get less pension.

My parents would then receive a half-pension,

they had a big problem.

I wanted to get rich ever since.

So that I could give them a good pension.

I have read books about becoming rich.

Listened to audiobooks.

Eventually, I came up with a financial system.

To systematically build up a fortune.

I have applied for a patent.

And I described the system in my first book:

How you build your own fortune with simple steps.

I have now published the 3rd edition of that book,

with the title Build your Fortune.

(I have received a patent on February 27th 2018.)

I could not find a job after that unemployment benefit.

I have emailed many job applications.

A lot employment agencies I visited.

In person I had visited with my resume,

more than 100 companies .

They did not have a job for me.

What could I do?

I did not want to go back to the hospitality industry anymore.

I liked investing a lot more.

So I started my first company

called Jasko,

on December 17, 2012

An investment company.

The saving and investing that I did for myself,

I could also do for other people.

I have had a realationship, a number of times

with a girl.

I fucked Hilde for the first time when I was 16.

Later I also have had sex with a girlfriend

of my mother .

Which is like 20 years older than me.

To be continued.

Are you looking forward to the sequel ?

It will be released on July 6th 2022

Note by november 22, 2020, ''You can read it on the following pages''

<u>book Victory III</u>

Hello Friend,
how are you ?

Is it strange that I say friend to you?
If you have bought and read Victory & Victory II,
and you also bought Victory III,
to read.
Then you put so much faith in me
as a friend does.

Thank you for being a loyal reader,
I really appreciate it.

I said the revenues (royalties)
from my books to the Giveth Life foundation,
and that from there more than 40 other Charities
receive donations.

So, by buying this book,
you now support them too,
more than 40 Charities.
Thanks & congratulations.

I really shouldn't be doing this …

But you have so much faith in me
I can show you.

It would be fine then
to prove to you,
what I say
also happens.

So I trust you

 **SNS**

44 2018, blad 2/6

Zakenrekening
NL09 SNSB 0705 9732 71

Date			Amount	Description
19-06	AF		0,25	PERIODIEKE OVERBOEKING NAAR NL73 INGB 0003 3377 37 stichting diva dichtbij Gift, hajrobv.nl
19-06	AF		0,25	PERIODIEKE OVERBOEKING NAAR NL54 RABO 0110 4360 08 voedselbank doetinchem Gift, hajrobv.nl
19-06	AF		0,25	PERIODIEKE OVERBOEKING NAAR NL68 RABO 0132 2355 36 Koninklijke nederlandse politiehondenvereniging Gift, hajrobv.nl
19-06	AF		0,25	PERIODIEKE OVERBOEKING NAAR NL49 RABO 0133 9780 95 stichting Joni Gift, hajrobv.nl
19-06	AF		0,25	PERIODIEKE OVERBOEKING NAAR NL25 RABO 0231 9575 48 VIOD Gift, hajrobv.nl
19-06	AF		0,25	PERIODIEKE OVERBOEKING NAAR NL14 ABNA 0533 4404 59 penningmeester S.V. doetinchem Gift, hajrobv.nl
19-06	BIJ		36,82	DE66 3006 0010 9999 9390 28 COTR0289089/4-DE66300600109999993 9028-KOBO INC PUBLISHER PAYMENTS (Acc.: KO1224)-ROYALTY PAYMENT WL00042062
20-06	AF		0,25	PERIODIEKE OVERBOEKING NAAR NL47 RABO 0312 3985 73 stichting vrienden van het Slingeland ziekenhuis Gift, hajrobv.nl
20-06	AF		0,25	PERIODIEKE OVERBOEKING NAAR NL23 RABO 0333 7779 99 kwf kankerbestrijding Gift, hajrobv.nl
20-06	AF		0,25	PERIODIEKE OVERBOEKING NAAR NL24 ABNA 0428 9798 15 stichting sportclub only friends Gift, hajrobv.nl
20-06	AF		5,00	PERIODIEKE OVERBOEKING NAAR NL42 RBRB 0919 2626 51 stichting laat het zieke kind genieten Gift, hajrobv.nl
20-06	AF		11,25	NL20 SNSB 8815 8669 14 STICHTING GIVETH LIFE
20-06	AF		18,41	NL20 SNSB 8815 8669 14 STICHTING GIVETH LIFE

You've seen a bank statement now
of the Giveth Life Foundation account number.
You see my book revenue (royalties)
paid out there on, by Kobo.

And you see evidence
that every day is donated to
Charities,
with modest amounts.
And monthly with a larger amount.

The donations,
that goes on every day & every month ...

I set it up like this
that it is automatic.

Because I am the founder & treasurer
of the Giveth Life foundation.

And you are now a donor &
supports more than 40 charities,
because you bought this book.

Wooohooo.

Together with you we support:

foundation Let the sick child enjoy, foundation Mini manna, Doctors without borders,
Kika, West Achterhoek Library, Association of nature monuments' s graveland,
Save the children, AAP foundation, Cliniclowns,
Achterhoek animal center, VIOD, Gasthuisfonds, Dierenlot foundation,
Royal Dutch Police Dog Association, Joni Foundation,
Chess Association doeinchem, NDD swimming club, Kidney Foundation,
Energy 4 all foundation, Cordaid, friends of the Slingeland hospital foundation,
foundation diva nearby, Kwf cancer prevention, foundation mama cash,
War Child, Chance Fund, Leprosy Foundation, Dutch Council for Refugees,
Food bank Doetincheem, Doetinchem hockey club, Free press unlimited
Orange Fund, Animal Protection, Mother Teresa Foundation
National MS fund, Noordbikers, Plan Nederland, Hartstichting,
Scouting the Netherlands fund, Unicef, Light for the world, Terre des hommes foundation,
Humanitas Association, Greenpeace Foundation, Opkikker Foundation, Children's Stamps Foundation,
Tuberculosis Fund, Baby Hope Foundation, UAF Foundation, Alzheimer Foundation,
Parkinson Fund, Thomas Aid Fund Madras, World Wildlife Fund, Street People Foundation,
Rudolph Foundation, V.V. Doetinchem, Youth Sports Fund Foundation
Amnesty International, Bartimeus Sonneheerdt association &
Disabled sports in the Netherlands.

This is how we contribute together,
to a better world.

Together we can give more.

Well maybe now you understand why you can purchase book Recipe for Happiness
. While you can also read it for free.
While it is the same book.

You can give the paid version as a gift,
but you also support more than 40 charities with it.
That's how you get a smug feeling,
by purchasing the paid version.

Ok, where did left of ?

So I would give the book Victory III to you .....

It will be about the past year,
So 2018.

And it should have some victories in it
to honor the title.

What victories…..

I made an Eshop for the Giveth Life foundation

you can visit it at:

https://eshopstichtinggivethlife.jimdofree.com/

I have done something different for once,
I made a video book.
Yes.

So a video in which I am on reading my 3rd book
Recipe for Happiness
to you.

Grab a nice cup of coffee or tea,
sit or lie down comfortably
and just play.

You can find video book at:

http://www.lulu.com/spotlight/jasminhajro

bottom left.

I also made a Hajro Group Photo Book.
I also made a Calendar for 2019,
you can also order them there.

(By now , 28 october 2020, Lulu has changed the author pages,
but you can still view my videobook at www.youtube.com)

I also made an author page
on Goodreads.

You can see it on:
https://www.goodreads.com/author/show/17686005.Jasmin_Hajro

I have also made some videos and put them on my author page
at Amazon.

You can see them on:

https://www.amazon.com/Jasmin-Hajro/e/B075GZPT4V

I've read some books of course,
because I want to get better at selling.

And I recommend them to you too.
They are :

Power of Self Confidence - Brian Tracy

Power of charm - Brian Tracy

21 great ways to become a sales superstar - B. Tracy

Stronger than ever - R. v / d Wolk

To sell is human - Daniel Pink

The secret of 100,000 - a year - L. Babeliowsky

I have also written and published some books,
and made some bundles (boxsets). And my ebooks can also be ordered as papeback.

book Website www.hajrobv.nl in a booklet

book the Lifebuoy for banks``loyal banking " (paperback)

book the Ultimate Winning Strategy for Entrepreneurs (ebook)

book Poems, jokes and book (paperback)

book Victory I.

book Victory II

book Always work & always money in your pocket, every day.

I have made a new edition of the book Double your profits.
(Double your Profits extended)

Book Things You Don't Want to Know
(I gave a copy of this to my dad for his birthday. Hopefully he can laugh about it)

book For you

My 14th book: starting your own business & making it successful,
in the harsh reality where nobody cares.

Bundle The largest, best & most spectacular book in the world

Bundle Double your profit & your bank balance in 4 months.

The bundles are collections of books ....
In Double your profit & your bank balance in 4 months
you get 5 books.
(The bundle does consist of 3 parts)

And bundle The grand, best & most spectacular
book in the world
is 11 books in 1.

That's a bargain right ...
You will then receive the entire Victorious series

My first series of books is that.

Thank you God for all the good things in my life.

I hope you don't mind
that I just said a prayer of thanks.

I am now writing the 3rd book of my SECOND series ...
(series Work to Shine)
I can be very grateful.

Thank you too for reading my writing.

And yes
it is 2:30 in the morning.

My little sister, the owner of Energie Nu &
the princess of which I am uncle (her daughter)
and her husband are still on vacation.
They will come back in 1 week.

My mother is still in a relationship with Peter,
and I am very happy for her that she has found a good person.

And I ?
Tjah still single.

First my life even better on track,
after that I'll find a wife.

Although I had the feeling a while ago
that I was dying.
It is a good & productive year after all...
We should be grateful.

Remember I would prove to you
that together we support many charities?
Here it comes.....

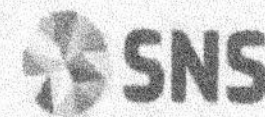

79 2018, blad 1/11

Vong saldo op 09-09-2018
€ 9,12 tegoed

Huidig saldo op 07-10-2018
€ **2,80** tekort

Zakenrekening
NL09 SNSB 0705 9732 71

10-09	AF	0,25	PERIODIEKE OVERBOEKING NAAR NL14 ABNA 0533 4404 59 penningmeester S.V. doetinchem Gift, hajrobv.nl
11-09	AF	0,25	PERIODIEKE OVERBOEKING NAAR NL11 RABO 0393 5867 66 Plan Nederland Gift, hajrobv.nl
11-09	BIJ	15,00	
11-09	AF	11,00	NL20 SNSB 8815 8669 14 STICHTING GIVETH LIFE
11-09	AF	0,25	EN Dividend 3 jarig bestaan Hajro

STICHTING GIVETH LIFE
Ottawastr 19
7007 BC DOETINCHEM

SNS Bank

Postbus 8466
3503 RL Utrecht

Vragen?
snsbank.nl/zakelijk
030 - 633 30 02

Op deze rekening is het depositogarantiestelsel van toepassing. Meer informatie leest u in het Informatieblad Depositogarantiestelsel op snsbank.nl/depositogarantiestelsel. Op uw verzoek sturen we u het Informatieblad Depositogarantiestelsel per post toe.

BIC SNSBNL2A

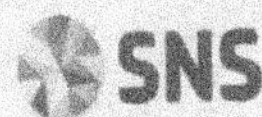

79 2018, blad 2/11

Zakenrekening
NL09 SNSB 0705 9732 71

11-09	AF	0,25	NL05 INGB 0003 9631 56 DIERENBESCHERMING Gift, 3 jarig bestaan Hajro (hajrobv.nl)
11-09	AF	1,58	Dekamarkt LOC527 DOETINCHE 11.09.2018 19U29 KV005 087N51 MCC:5411
11-09	AF	8,10	Dekamarkt LOC527 DOETINCHE 11.09.2018 19U32 KV005 0JDM1V MCC:5411
12-09	AF	0,25	PERIODIEKE OVERBOEKING NAAR NL96 INGB 0006 0596 89 stichting artrose Gift, hajrobv.nl
12-09	AF	0,25	PERIODIEKE OVERBOEKING NAAR NL74 ABNA 0707 0702 52 save the children Gift, hajrobv.nl
12-09	BIJ	20,00	
12-09	AF	2,05	NL20 SNSB 8815 8669 14 STICHTING GIVETH LIFE
12-09	AF	1,00	NL20 SNSB 8815 8669 14 STICHTING GIVETH LIFE
12-09	AF	8,77	Kruidvat 6145 DOETINCHE 12.09.2018 15U49 KV005 C9FRD2 MCC:5331
12-09	AF	3,69	Action 1063 Doetinche 12.09.2018 15U58 KV005 72145977 MCC:5310
13-09	AF	0,25	PERIODIEKE OVERBOEKING NAAR NL64 INGB 0002 7775 30 stichting AAP Gift, hajrobv.nl
14-09	AF	0,25	PERIODIEKE OVERBOEKING NAAR NL31 INGB 000D 0066 40 stichting Cliniclowns Gift, hajrobv.nl
15-09	AF	0,25	PERIODIEKE OVERBOEKING NAAR NL13 RABO 0117 3974 66 stichting kanjers voor kanjers Gift, hajrobv.nl
15-09	AF	0,25	PERIODIEKE OVERBOEKING NAAR NL57 RABO 0154 3412 58 stichting Dierencentrum achterhoek Gift, hajrobv.nl
15-09	AF	0,25	PERIODIEKE OVERBOEKING NAAR NL85 RABO 0192 0849 09 stichting speciaal onderwijs Gift, hajrobv.nl

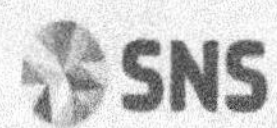 **SNS**

15-09	AF	0,25	PERIODIEKE OVERBOEKING NAAR NL85 RABO 0192 0849 09 stichting speciaal onderwijs Gift, hajrobv.nl
15-09	AF	0,25	PERIODIEKE OVERBOEKING NAAR NL93 ABNA 0230 7087 30 stichting lucas onderwijs Gift, hajrobv.nl
15-09	BIJ	6,00	NL20 SNSB 8815 8669 14 STICHTING GIVETH LIFE
15-09	AF	5,74	Action 1063 Doetinche 15.09.2018 15U01 KV005 72146046 MCC:5310
16-09	AF	0,25	PERIODIEKE OVERBOEKING NAAR NL28 INGB 0000 0023 29 stichting Dierenlot Gift, hajrobv.nl
17-09	AF	0,25	PERIODIEKE OVERBOEKING NAAR NL96 INGB 0000 0044 03 stichting energy 4 all Gift, hajrobv.nl
17-09	AF	0,25	PERIODIEKE OVERBOEKING NAAR NL73 INGB 0003 3377 37 stichting diva dichtbij Gift, hajrobv.nl
17-09	BIJ	5,00	
17-09	BIJ	22,50	
17-09	BIJ	37,19	DE66 3006 0010 9999 9390 28 COTRO309100/38-DE663006001099999 39028-KOBO INC PUBLISHER PAYMENT S (Acc.: KO1224)-ROYALTY PAYMENT WL00042062
17-09	AF	42,00	Bestelling Hajro
17-09	AF	10,00	Vergoeding bezorgen voor Hajro
17-09	AF	2,05	NL54 RABO 0110 4360 08 VOEDSELBANK DOETINCHEM Gift 3 jarig bestaan Hajro
17-09	AF	2,05	NL90 INGB 0003 2045 41 STICHTING MINI MANNA Gift 3 jarig bestaan Hajro
17-09	AF	2,00	NL20 SNSB 8815 8669 14 STICHTING GIVETH LIFE
18-09	AF	5,00	PERIODIEKE OVERBOEKING NAAR Gebruik zakelijke ruimte door Ha jro, inclusief huur, electra, wa ter, internet etc

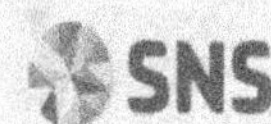 **SNS**

18-09	AF	0,25	PERIODIEKE OVERBOEKING NAAR NL09 RABO 0157 5822 13 Stichting Jeugdsportfonds Gelderland Gift, hajrobv.nl
18-09	BIJ	20,00	
18-09	AF	5,00	NL20 SNSB 8815 8669 14 STICHTING GIVETH LIFE
18-09	AF	0,35	NL70 INGB 0000 0880 00 NIERSTICHTING Gift 3 jarig bestaan Hajro
18-09	AF	8,10	Dekamarkt LOC527 DOETINCHE 18.09.2018 18U30 KV005 0QZ817 MCC:5411
19-09	AF	0,25	PERIODIEKE OVERBOEKING NAAR NL49 RABO 0133 9780 95 stichting Joni Gift, hajrobv.nl
20-09	AF	0,25	PERIODIEKE OVERBOEKING NAAR NL89 INGB 0000 0081 18 Stichting Kinderen Kankervrij Gift, hajrobv.nl
20-09	BIJ	20,00	
20-09	AF	11,80	Action 1063 Doetinche 20.09.2018 14U06 KV005 72146046 MCC:5310
21-09	AF	0,25	PERIODIEKE OVERBOEKING NAAR NL42 RBRB 0919 2626 51 stichting laat het zieke kind genieten Gift, hajrobv.nl
21-09	BIJ	30,00	
21-09	AF	25,00	Gebruik zakelijke ruimte door Ha jro, inclusief huur, electra, wa ter, internet etc
22-09	AF	0,25	PERIODIEKE OVERBOEKING NAAR NL58 INGB 0000 0005 28 stichting mama cash Gift, hajrobv.nl
23-09	AF	0,25	PERIODIEKE OVERBOEKING NAAR NL90 INGB 0003 2045 41 stichting Mini manna Gift, hajrobv.nl
24-09	AF	0,25	PERIODIEKE OVERBOEKING NAAR NL31 ABNA 0533 0178 15 stichting vrienden van het Slingeland ziekenhuis Gift, hajrobv.nl

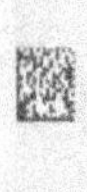

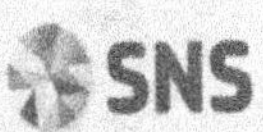 **SNS**

24-09	Bij	35,00	
24-09	Bij	35,00	
24-09	Bij	23,00	
24-09	AF	12,00	NL20 SNSB 8815 8669 14 STICHTING GIVETH LIFE
24-09	AF	25,00	NL40 RABO 0350 8011 93 6720180924 0020002099644713 iDEA L jongerius.nl
			Referentie: 2018- 09-24 11:57 002000209964471
24-09	AF	9,64	Action 1063 Doetinche 24.09.2018 13U31 KV005 72146046 MCC:5310
24-09	AF	3,63	Dekamarkt LOC527 DOETINCHE 24.09.2018 13U37 KV005 087N51 MCC:5411
24-09	AF	16,88	Dekamarkt LOC527 DOETINCHE 24.09.2018 13U40 KV005 00Z817 MCC:5411
24-09	Bij	0,25	Opdracht met tegenrekening NL31A BNA0533017815 kon niet worden ui tgevoerd.
			Reden: Rekening is opg eheven
25-09	AF	25,00	PERIODIEKE OVERBOEKING NAAR NL45 INGB 0005 1133 41 Yards 8253471
25-09	AF	5,00	PERIODIEKE OVERBOEKING NAAR Gebruik
			zakelijke ruimte door Ha jro, inclusief huur, electra, wa ter, internet etc
25-09	AF	0,25	PERIODIEKE OVERBOEKING NAAR NL25 RABO 0231 9575 48 VIOD Gift, hajrobv.nl
25-09	AF	10,00	PERIODIEKE OVERBOEKING NAAR NL82 ABNA 0636 7419 07 Managementboek.nl
			Studieboeken Hajro / J. Hajro
25-09	AF	1,08	MAANDELIJKSE KOSTEN WERELDPAS KAARTNR. 005 TEN NAME VAM
26-09	AF	0,25	PERIODIEKE OVERBOEKING NAAR NL44 RABO 0157 1826 22 stichting opkikker Gift,
			hajrobv.nl
26-09	Bij	50,00	

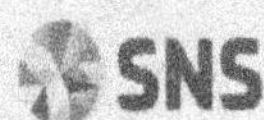 **SNS**

26-09	AF	16,67	NL06 COBA 0637 0537 53 Europese incasso door:TELE2 NEDE RLAND B.V.
			NL-ARNLNL1812986629-I ncassant ID: NL12T2N333034180000 -Kenmerk Machtiging:
			B0008075774 -0705973271-01-ARNLNL1812986629
26-09	AF	10,00	vakantie vergoeding, werkzaamhed en
			Hajro
26-09	AF	10,00	vergoeding, bezorgen voor Hajro
26-09	Bij	27,00	NL20 SNSB 8815 8669 14 STICHTING GIVETH LIFE
26-09	AF	45,00	Gebruik zakelijke ruimte door Ha jro,
			inclusief huur, electra, wa ter, internet etc
26-09	AF	0,25	NL14 ABNA 0533 4404 59 PENNINGMEESTER S.V. DOETINCHEM Gift 3 jarig bestaan Hajro
26-09	AF	0,25	NL14 ABNA 0533 4404 59 PENNINGMEESTER S.V. DOETINCHEM Gift, Hajro
			(www.hajrobv.nl)
27-09	AF	0,25	PERIODIEKE OVERBOEKING NAAR NL47 RABO 0312 3985 73 Stichting Vrienden Slingeland
			Ziekenhuis Gift, hajro (hajrobv.nl)
27-09	AF	0,25	PERIODIEKE OVERBOEKING NAAR NL10 ABNA 0504 2015 30 stichting parkinsonfonds
			Gift, hajrobv.nl
27-09	Bij	10,00	
28-09	AF	0,28	PERIODIEKE OVERBOEKING NAAR NL13 INGB 0000 0025 02 alzheimer nederland Gift,
			hajrobv.nl
28-09	AF	0,25	NL32 TRIO 0197 8537 57 STICHTING PRESENT DOETINCHEM Gift, hajrobv.nl
28-09	AF	0,25	NL75 RABO 0314 3726 01 SPEELTUIN ONTSPANNING VERENIGING Gift, hajrobv.nl
28-09	AF	2,55	NL20 SNSB 8815 8669 14 STICHTING GIVETH LIFE

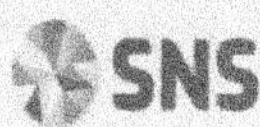

SNS

79 2018, blad 7/11

Zakenrekening
NL09 SNSB 0705 9732 71

29-09	AF	0,35	PERIODIEKE OVERBOEKING NAAR NL31 INGB 0000 0066 40 stichting Cliniclowns Gift, hajrobv.nl
29-09	AF	5,00	PERIODIEKE OVERBOEKING NAAR NL28 INGB 0006 7498 43 ING
30-09	AF	0,25	PERIODIEKE OVERBOEKING NAAR NL84 INGB 0000 0505 00 leprastichting Gift, hajrobv.nl
30-09	AF	0,25	PERIODIEKE OVERBOEKING NAAR NL61 RABO 0157 2075 36 stichting sport en reacreatie Gift, hajrobv.nl
01-10	AF	0,25	PERIODIEKE OVERBOEKING NAAR NL18 INGB 0000 0008 60 hersenstichting Gift, hajrobv.nl
01-10	AF	0,45	PERIODIEKE OVERBOEKING NAAR NL94 INGB 0004 0040 40 vereniging Bartimeus sonneheerdt Gift, hajrobv.nl
01-10	AF	0,25	PERIODIEKE OVERBOEKING NAAR NL68 RABO 0132 2355 36 Koninklijke nederlandse politiehondenvereniging Gift, hajrobv.nl
01-10	AF	0,25	PERIODIEKE OVERBOEKING NAAR NL92 ABNA 0924 0654 27 St. Bibliotheek West Achterhoek Gift, hajrobv.nl
01-10	BIJ	5,00	
01-10	BIJ	5,00	- Cadeau mok
01-10	BIJ	0,10	GB51 DEUT 4050 8127 3042 11 OFA000123618368-GB51DEUT40508127 304211-AMAZON MEDIA EU SARL-Paym ent.: 81946876 null
02-10	AF	0,25	PERIODIEKE OVERBOEKING NAAR NL13 INGB 0000 0040 54 artsen zonder grenzen Gift, hajrobv.nl
02-10	AF	5,00	PERIODIEKE OVERBOEKING Gebruik zakelijke ruimte door Ha jro, inclusief huur, electra, wa ter, internet etc

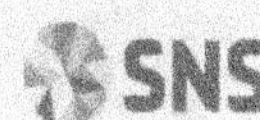

SNS

79 2018, blad 8/11

Zakenrekening
NL09 SNSB 0705 9732 71

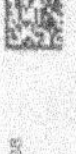

02-10	AF	0,25	PERIODIEKE OVERBOEKING NAAR NL67 RABO 0148 5814 12 Stichting Ontmoetinchem Gift, hajrobv.nl
02-10	BIJ	25,00	
02-10	BIJ	5,00	
02-10	BIJ	0,06	GB62 DEUT 4050 8127 3042 07 OFA000123444463-GB62DEUT40508127 304207-AMAZON MEDIA EU SARL-Paym ent.: 81710204 null
02-10	AF	21,94	NL51 ABNA 0565 6686 25 1615384885302004 003000327460381 1 13514950 Lulu Referentie: 2018 -10-02 15:56 003000327460381
02-10	AF	3,84	Action 1063 Doetinche 2.10.2018 16U09 KV005 72146046 MCC:5310
02-10	AF	6,60	Dekamarkt LOC527 DOETINCHE 2.10.2018 16U12 KV005 0QZ817 MCC:5411
02-10	AF	1,68	Dekamarkt LOC527 DOETINCHE 2.10.2018 19U04 KV005 087N51 MCC:5411
03-10	AF	0,25	PERIODIEKE OVERBOEKING NAAR NL57 INGB 0000 0009 34 Cordaid Gift, hajrobv.nl
03-10	AF	0,25	PERIODIEKE OVERBOEKING NAAR NL95 INGB 0000 0550 55 longfonds Gift, hajrobv.nl
03-10	AF	1,00	PERIODIEKE OVERBOEKING NAAR Dividend Hajro
03-10	AF	1,00	PERIODIEKE OVERBOEKING NAAR Energie Nu Dividend Hajro
03-10	AF	0,25	PERIODIEKE OVERBOEKING NAAR NL17 RABO 0311 3002 00 Gehandicaptensport Nederland Gift, hajrobv.nl
03-10	BIJ	5,00	NL28 INGB 0006 7498 43 370018457994-NL28INGB0006749843- Nationale-Nederlanden-uw betalin g 01/10/2018. n
03-10	AF	0,35	NL38 RABO 0384 3711 83 STICHTING SPINDO Gift Hajro, (hajrobv.nl)
03-10	AF	0,25	NL38 RABO 0384 3711 83 STICHTING SPINDO Gift 3 jarig bestaan Hajro
04-10	AF	0,25	PERIODIEKE OVERBOEKING NAAR NL05 INGB 0003 9631 56 Dierenbescherming Gift, hajrobv.nl

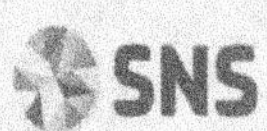 **SNS**

04-10	AF	0,25	PERIODIEKE OVERBOEKING NAAR NL56 RABO 0166 3663 66 war child Gift, hajrobv.nl
04-10	AF	1,00	PERIODIEKE OVERBOEKING NAAR NL22 Dividend Hajro
04-10	AF	1,00	PERIODIEKE OVERBOEKING NAAR NL81 Dividend Hajro
04-10	AF	1,00	PERIODIEKE OVERBOEKING NAAR NL83 Dividend Hajro
04-10	BIJ	22,00	NL88 RABO 0327 9238 49
04-10	AF	5,41	Action 1063 Doetinche 4.10.2018 15U27 KV005 72145977 MCC:5310
04-10	AF	3,96	Dekamarkt LOC527 DOETINCHE 4.10.2018 15U32 KV005 087N51 MCC:5411
05-10	AF	0,25	PERIODIEKE OVERBOEKING NAAR NL58 INGB 0000 0057 66 diabetes fonds Gift, hajrobv.nl
05-10	AF	0,25	PERIODIEKE OVERBOEKING NAAR NL60 INGB 0000 1234 88 vluchtelingenwerk nederland Gift, hajrobv.nl
05-10	AF	0,25	PERIODIEKE OVERBOEKING NAAR NL17 RABO 0311 3002 00 Gehandicaptensport Nederland Gift, hajrobv.nl
05-10	AF	0,50	PERIODIEKE OVERBOEKING NAAR NL38 RABO 0384 3711 83 stichting Spindo Gift Hajro, (hajrobv.nl)
05-10	BIJ	24,00	
05-10	AF	4,99	Kruidvat 6145 DOETINCHE 5.10.2018 20U32 KV005 C9FRD2 MCC:5331
05-10	AF	3,00	NL20 SNSB 8815 8669 14 STICHTING GIVETH LIFE
05-10	AF	0,25	NL11 RABO 0195 2732 73 STICHTING KLEDINGBANK DOETINCHEM Gift Hajro (www.hajrobv.nl)
05-10	AF	0,35	NL11 RABO 0195 2732 73 STICHTING KLEDINGBANK DOETINCHEM Gift 3 jarig bestaan Hajro
05-10	AF	0,25	NL86 RABO 0134 1384 49 VRIENDEN VAN ELVER STICHTING Gift Hajro (www.hajrobv.nl)

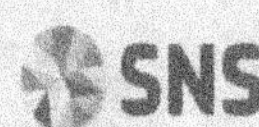 **SNS**

79 2018, blad 10/11

Zakenrekening
NLog SNSB 0705 9732 71

05-10	AF	0,25	NL50 INGB 0000 1000 00 STICHTING ALS Gift Hajro (www.hajrobv.nl)
06-10	AF	0,25	PERIODIEKE OVERBOEKING NAAR NL83 INGB 0000 2221 11 epilepsi fonds Gift, hajrobv.nl
06-10	AF	0,25	PERIODIEKE OVERBOEKING NAAR NL54 RABO 0110 4360 08 voedselbank doetinchem Gift, hajrobv.nl
06-10	AF	0,25	PERIODIEKE OVERBOEKING NAAR NL70 RABO 0142 1730 53 stichting Jeugdsportfonds Gift, hajrobv.nl
06-10	AF	0,25	PERIODIEKE OVERBOEKING NAAR NL41 INGB 0675 8622 05 Kansfonds Gift, hajrobv.nl
06-10	AF	6,66	Dekamarkt LOC527 DOETINCHE 6.10.2018 20U44 KV005 087N51 MCC:5411
07-10	AF	0,25	PERIODIEKE OVERBOEKING NAAR NL92 INGB 0000 0076 76 free press unlimited Gift, hajrobv.nl
07-10	AF	0,25	PERIODIEKE OVERBOEKING NAAR NL86 RABO 0134 1384 49 vrienden van Elver stichting Gift, hajrobv.nl
07-10	AF	0,45	PERIODIEKE OVERBOEKING NAAR NL11 RABO 0195 2732 73 stichting Kledingbank doetinchem Gift, hajrobv.nl
07-10	AF	0,25	PERIODIEKE OVERBOEKING NAAR NL45 TRIO 0198 1000 00 Amnesty International Gift, hajrobv.nl
07-10	AF	0,25	PERIODIEKE OVERBOEKING NAAR NL23 RABO 0333 7779 99 kwf kankerbestrijding Gift, hajrobv.nl
07-10	AF	0,25	PERIODIEKE OVERBOEKING NAAR NL61 RABO 0370 0252 45 doetinchemse hockey club Gift, hajrobv.nl
07-10	AF	0,25	PERIODIEKE OVERBOEKING NAAR NL83 ABNA 0447 2694 61 stichting Friends indeed Gift, hajrobv.nl

Some names and numbers have been left out,
for privacy.

I hope you can read it ...

Otherwise you can still view it at:
https://www.hajrobv.nl/doen-wat-je-zegt-of-schrijf

And what about that patent?

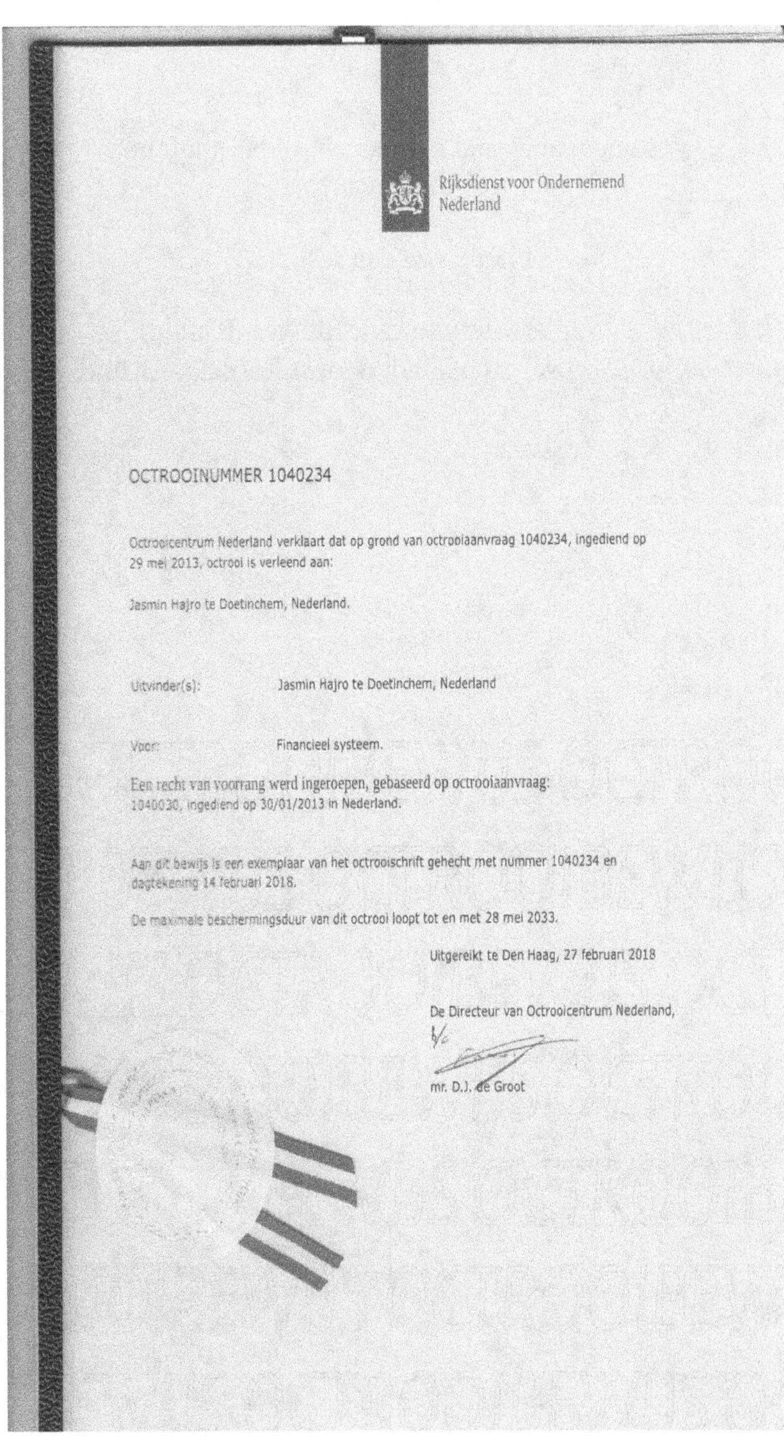

I have described that financial system in
my book How to Build Your Own Fortune with Simple Steps (2nd edition)
& in the 3rd edition, namely book Build your Fortune.

I really recommend that you buy that book,
and take the steps
contained in it.

Am I our 'hero'?
I don't know if I did anything heroic.

But I did do something spectacular
maybe it is Legendary ....

The following :

One of the goals of company Hajro is
doing something back for the Netherlands.
Because the founder of Hajro
(also called Jasko)
is an immigrant &
was well received in the Netherlands by the Dutch.

Because his book Build your Fortune
(what every household should have)
is available free of charge to everyone in the Netherlands.
To build a fortune or
a good pension.
Hajro Achieved This Goal!

You can also read that on my homepage:
www.hajrobv.nl

I have achieved one of my Long-term Goals.
Great huh?

I'm very happy.

As you can see it's almost 3 in the morning
when I wake up & get up in the morning in the morning
may it be called a miracle.
So I still struggle a bit with getting up early.

After this I also have to publish this book,
so it will be later.

I still smoke too much black tabacco &
drink more coffee than is good for me.

But yes, you gotta die from something right ?.

A week on the road with me (in short)

I have from Sunday September 2, 2018 to
Saturday, September 15
worked every day.

Every day I started selling door to door for a long time.
With sets of greeting cards & gift mugs.

And I have found 47 customers
times 5 euros that is
235 euros in turnover.

I bought a birthday present for my sister.
I gave my nephew a Quest magazine as a gift.
(who lives in Assen)
I paid my deliverer the fee.
I bought Mary Kay hand cream as a gift
for my mom.

That Sunday after those 2 weeks,
I was tired but satisfied.
I then rested & watched movies.

I had worked in city Doetinchem and on Sunday in town Didam.

Another victory
I made 103 sales in September,
my new record.
(meaning I found 103 customers)

That is 515 euros in turnover,
plus 37, - in royalties
of book sales.

I'm lucky to still live with my mother.

But I'm already halfway there.
When I make 200 sales per month,
I can basically look for a house.

My mother is a person of gold.

I'm going to earn a ton (100,000 euros)
and then again.
Then I will buy a house for my mom
and a car (a purple one)

Are you also going to do something spectacular for your parents?

They are always there for you

I hope you enjoyed
and that I have kept my word on what I promised.

Victory IV

For my mother Azema Halilovic ...
Thank you draga majko (dear mother)
that you are always there for me.
And that you gave me the time to build my company
& to write so many books.

Victory IV

Hey Hello
how are you doing ?
In principle, I'm fine ... yet it is a bit mixed ...
it is Monday, April 20, 2020.
it's been 2 months Corona time ..
just a fucking flu ..
old people with poor resistance die from the flu.
Our neighbor has passed away, he had bad lungs for years.
I worked anyway ... all this time…
It's harder ... it takes much longer to find a customer and I face more closed doors.
I found 3 today, 3 customers ...
who have bought a set of our unique greeting cards …
I designed them myself and only we have them, so they are unique.

''Note at the time of translation, Sunday november 22, I am human too, I could be wrong''

We have a temporary promotion ... or offer…
the well known buy one, get one free...
if you buy a set of greeting cards, then you get a giftmug for free.
To cheer the people up a bit, in this "strange time" ".
Maybe you got on the news that some businesses and shops are closed,
re was talk of lockdowns of countries, they want people to keep their distance from each
other and in the supermarket the cashier was wearing gloves.
he paper said that if you didn't have any symptoms of a cold for 24 hours, you just got
over it and you are fine...
I have written 2 booklets in recent times ...
For Saartje
and Secrets of writing and selling books.
ue to current government measures I did get a Tozo ... which is corona crisis subsidy…
Hoeray finally financial support from the government ..
the money is of course nice,

but above all it is the principle ...
It means... we do not pay taxes for nothing.
Because if you need help, you will get it ... apparently ..
even if it just took a long time for me to get some.
And only after my 6th application for benefits, the Tozo subsidy got approved.
Dutch government and tax authorities …
Thank you.
I don't feel like a 2nd class citizen anymore.

With more than 36 books and
still no bestseller …
I start to wonder if I am doing something wrong?
What do you think ?
But I know what it is ...
Marketing ...
I have to do more marketing ...
maybe several thousand people know that I write books
and where you can buy my books ...
In a world of more than 6 billion people ….a several thousand is not so much people…
I also write in my diary ...

my journal ...
a little less than I used to do lately ...
I was busy…
so I wrote those 2 books ...
I have worked..
selling our greeting cards ...
I also made Author Merchandise ….maybe you think that's cool or nice ..
Tshirt with "Victorious" on it
or "Work to shine"
like my book series ...
and ofcourse also "" You legend "

and an author mug
And a Tshirt with a funny but true text:
" My poo is black from all the coffee. I am a writer "
Wouldn't it be funny to walk around with that ...
In addition, also a Tshirt with the logo from my company Hajro
and a sweater which is also printed with our logo.
You can see them all at www.gumroad.com/jasminhajro
I have made and delivered mix sets to our Member,

a customer of mine who has a greeting card subscription,
every month she receives greeting cards with something extra.
And I also have working links put on my Author website,
if you click on it then you actually end up on the website of the bookstores
where my books are for sale.
It all takes time to do and create and energy ..
Maybe that's why I was a little tired the past few days..
I hadn't even thought about it ...
And I also added Marketing for Author as a service to my company's services.
Because that's what I and other book authors need.
what I do for myself I can also do as a business for other people.
Beethoven plays in the background while I write ...
I like classical music ...

''Note by the time of translation, november 22nd 2020, my company's website is www.hajro.be
I have paid for it a year upfront….so it's always online and working…
I have a new Author website...whaich has a longass domain name…..but it's free and always online,
avilable for you to visit and ofcourse online 24/7…..I give away 10 of my books on it….so it's
worth a visit…..just remember the longass domain name which is
www.jasminhajro6.webnode.nl   ''

This is one of the unique

greetingcards, which is

in a package of 5

greetingcards and

envelopes,

that I sell.

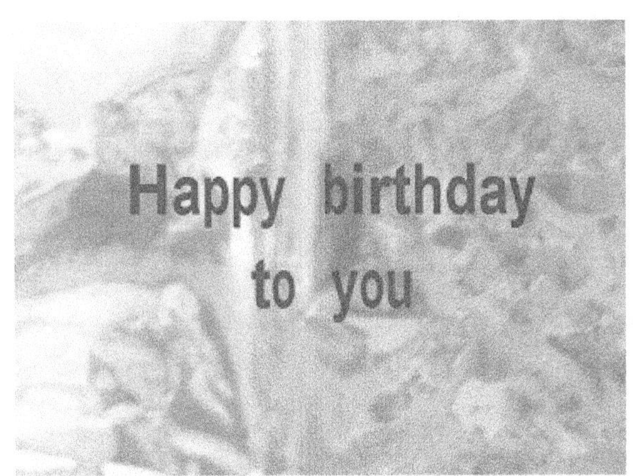

(I have sold more than 700 of these packages of greetingcards)

And this is the giftmug, full of candy

that people get along with the package of greetingcards for free,

for a limited time

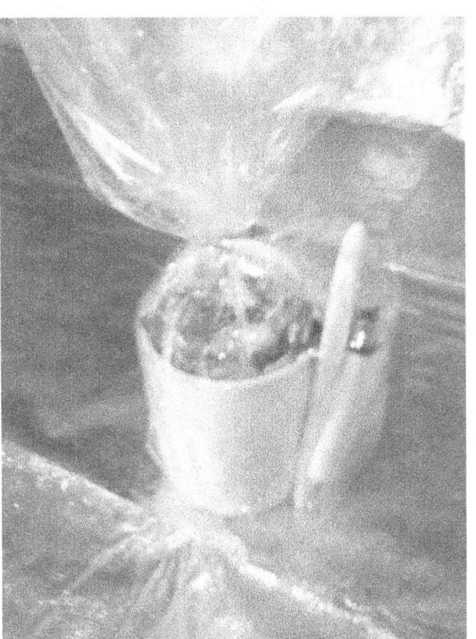

The mug has my company's logo printed on it and it also says : ''Enjoy life''

I was thinking of writing a fiction book
a kind of "rant"
" swearing on things I hate or to blow off steam ...
as to "pickers" or pluckers...
" too lazy to work want something for free ... living of other people by theft ...
drug other people to pick them better ...
What do you think ?
Is it gonna be a weird fucking book?
Should I just stay in my arena …
my box the NONfiction area….

I respect working people ...
I like to work .. working has positively changed my life ...
I know how hard some people have to work for their money
... I respect that ...
I jogged this afternoon ... it was going slow ...
it has been a while since my last run... 1 or maybe 2 weeks ago

that I was last running ..
scandalous I know…
I jogged a lot more in the past year ...
I have to get back into the habit of running regularly.

Sometimes I would like it to come back to someone at home after work…
I'm alone for a long time ..
I just haven't actively looked for a relationship ...
I first wanted to get my life in order ...
It's more or less in order ...
I do not drink I don't use ..
I don't make any problems ..
I work…
Ready?
Ready for a relationship?
First I'll have to earn a normal ... minimum of E 1500, - per month.

Then at least I can do nice things with my woman..
.. good food and stuff
and go to the McDonalds of course ...
But also because it gives peace, when everything is paid.

''Another note, by the time of translation ….

I know it's short…
I don't like that either…
I don't want to disappoint you….

It's just that I've been so busy..
building my business…
designing new greetingcards….
Adding new products and services…

and then I had to create a new company website
and also a new author website…

And when the corona crisis began…
I had to do something to keep my business going…
like the promotion…
buy one, get one free…

I had to Apply for subsidy and funding…

en I decided that the best way to get through the crisis was..
to just keep on working…
so I kept on selling door to door my greetingcards..

and I wrote more books…

Sometimes I worked 6 or 7 days a week…
and on my free day I would visit my sister and her kids…
the girl is 2 years old now and the boy is 1 year old and he just started to walk...

Here they are…
my books of this crisis year…

Through the crisis english
Running out of time
In loving memory
Actie als strategie
Rahima & Idriz
Exposium
Hajro, story & catalogus
My story english
Word miljonair in sales
Wat het beste werkt ? na 7 jaar ondernemen
Ondernemen met hersenschadE
Productiviteit crash course

And I also translated Victory 3 into english…
and now also Victory 4…

By november I got like exhausted…
and took 3 to 4 days off every week….

And…
well guess what..?

I also wrote ''My little masterpiece''
I recommend you get that one..
the booklet has a great quote for everyday of the month..
they are things you can do…
and they are lifechanging…
for sale at : My little masterpiece (lulu.com)

Ans after that I wrote : I don't feel like writing, says the author
it's more of a whitepaper…
but it's still valuable…
for sale at : I don't feel like writing says the author (lulu.com)

These 2 booklets I have written in english
it saves me the time of translating them…

On the following pages you can read my booklets…
the Recipe for Happiness
and
Overcoming tough times…

or if you have already read them..
you can reread them…
and find something of value …
that you didn't see
the first time…

<u>Recipe for happiness</u>

In this short booklet you will discover:

The bio of author Jasmin Hajro

&

book The Recipe for Happiness :

Introduction,

Chapter I,

Chapter II,

Note from the author.

&

A preview of book Build Your Fortune

&

A small acquaintance with establishment Hajro

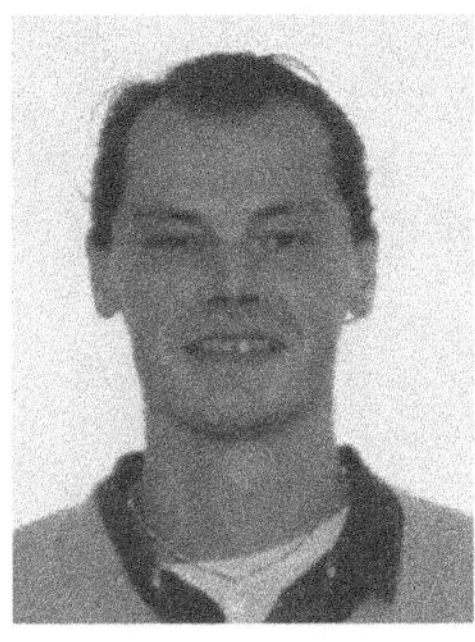

Hello dear reader,

how are you ?

Thank you for buying booklet Recipe for Happiness.

My name is Jasmin Hajro, I was born on July 6, 1985 in Bosnia.

As refugees, we came to the Netherlands 21 years ago.

After having completed school & worked at several jobs ...

n 17 December 2012, I founded my first company: investment firm Jasko.

After a successful first year, I unfortunately had to close that company.

After a short period of rest, unemployment and temporary work.

I started again as an entrepreneur.

On September 1, 2015, I founded establishment Hajro.

(We say establishment instead of company,

because we do a bit more then just sell stuff.

Like providing jobs,

donating to 40 different charities,

and helping people to live richer.)

Since the beginning the core activity is,

selling sets of greeting cards, door to door.

Nowadays the product range has been expanded.

With, among other things, the selling of my 10 books.

The royalties of my books are donated

to the charity: foundation Giveth Life.

My company is now part of Hajro Group,

which consists of 20 different subsidiaries,

that are part of 1 umbrella organization.

For more information about my company &

the foundation, go to my website : www.hajrobv.nl

The Recipe for Happiness, introduction

A book has been written about a true story ...

About a man who was imprisoned in a concentration camp

at the time of Hitler,

and happy.

So,

Happiness has nothing to do with your circumstances.

It has everything to do with,

your choice to be happy,

regardless of circumstances.

Choose to be happy.

Of course there are touhger times in life,

like when someone you love,

dies.

That's part of life.

Those times of grief you just have to go through and process.

Processing is best done by talking about it,

to get it off your chest regularly.

Or by writing about it,

if you write down a situation or your feelings about it,

then it's on paper,

and it is less in your head.

Writing is a good outlet.

Processing is also done well by:

staying busy.

Whether that is in your work or your hobby.

They say: a rolling stone does not collect moss.

So stay busy ....

Okay, now you have learned a good lesson about how to

better process negative life experiences.

But you're here for the Recipe for Happiness, right?

Well, the lesson you've learned will help to
make the recipe work better for you.

<u>Chapter I</u>

Here it comes then ...

You have probably read a local newspaper,
and you regularly check the news.

(the daily news on television)

Have you noticed that about 99% of it is bad news?
Only misery ..
If you did not know better,
you would think that the whole world is going to perish.

If it's a habit for you,
to watch the news every day for half an hour ...

Have you ever wondered if it's healthy for you?
Does it make you happy ?

Of course not !

The easiest way to change a habit is

by replacing it with a new habit.

So from today on,

instead of watching the worldly news

half an hour a day ....

Watch COMEDY for half an hour a day.

Mandatory.

Every day.

Well, now at half past eight in the evening it's not news time,

but Comedy time.

If you watch comedy,

you relax &

you laugh.

Sounds healthier, doesn't it?

Well, laughing every day is easy to do, right?

And replacing your old bad habit in this way,

with a nice, healthy new habit,

is probably easier than you thought.

Except that relaxation is good for you,

when you laugh,

your body makes endorphins.

Those are natural happiness substances.

Well, after 21 days of daily watching comedy,

you will have formed a new habit.

So watch Comedy every day.

You can watch a lot of standup comedy on Youtube for free.

Simple?

Sure, but you have to do it,

every day,

until you don't have to think about it anymore,

and you start doing it automatically.

<u>Chapter II</u>

Some Happiness Ingredients in a row:

- Watch comedy every day, at least one hour.

- Eat ice cream, treat someone with an ice cream.

- Work out, throw out your frustration by playing tennis

or go for a run.

—   Pee in the yard

(and if you get a fine for urinating, laugh your ass off)

—   Do not worry, life is too short for that

(by staying busy, you do not have time to worry)

—   Hug the people that you love

—   Go enjoy a cup of coffee or tea

—   Buy or save a cat or some other pet

—   When you receive money, immediately save a part of it

—   Don't let the media scare you,

the world is not getting worse, the world is getting better.

—   Sex, need I say more

(when you have sex your body also produces endorphins =

those natural happiness substances)

Maybe the Recipe for Happiness

is different than you had expected....

But that doesn't matter,

the point is that it works &

that it will help you to live happier.

Do it,

it is easier

then looking with a sour face.

<u>Note from the author</u>

If you liked this book & got some value from it.

Would you then be so kind,

please,

to recommend it

to the people that you know.

So that they too can enjoy it

and live happier.

Thank you very much.

____

It was my pleasure to write and translate

this book (my third one) for you.

I hope it helps you to live happier.

(I know it will, if you do the things it teaches)

And I hope, that we can together make a contribution

to more happiness in the world.

We can.
If you recommend this book
and share it.
Then I will promote it.

And together we will make a contribution to

a happier world.

I would appreciate it if you would write a short review.
Thank you for your effort.

Kind regards,

Jasmin Hajro

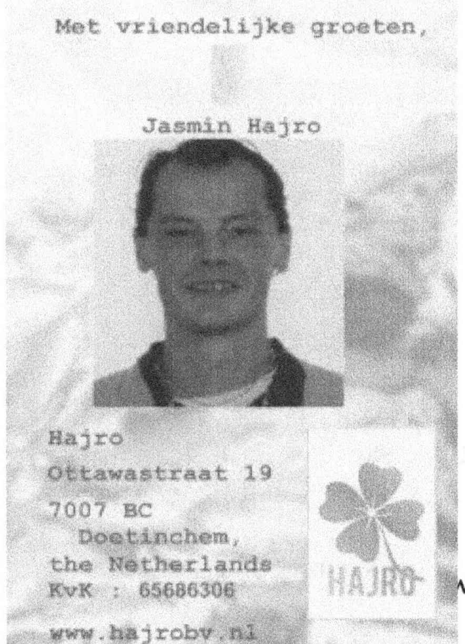

w Jouw Fortuin

Preview book Build your fortune

<u>the Pay yourself first principle</u>

It means that when you receive your money,
you first pay yourself, by for example, setting aside a tenth.

To clarify your result,
we will make an example calculation.

For example, you earn 3000 euros or dollars per month.
And you pay yourself first,
in other words: you put aside a tenth (10%) of your income.
So you save 300, - euros per month.

A year has 12 months,
So after 1 year you'll have (12 x 300) = 3600, - euros.
After 1 year you have put a whole month's salary aside.

If you put aside a tenth every month,
how much will you have after 10 years?

(3600 x 10) = 36000, - euro.
So after 10 years you have 36000 euros
or a whole year's salary in your saving account.

Later on in this book: Build your Fortune,
you'll see how to make
that amount that you put aside each month.
Grow faster.

Preview book Build your Fortune

<u>10% of everything</u>

It is important that when you first pay yourself,
by setting aside 10%.
That you put 10% of everything aside.

Of course 10% of your income.

But also 10% of the tips if you receive any,

also 10% of your surtax,

also 10% of the money you receive as a gift,

also 10% of your 13th month,

also 10% of your bonus,

also 10% of your wage increase,

also 10% of your tax refund,

also 10% of your welcome bonus,

also 10% of your holidaypay.

No matter from which angle or from whom you receive money,
the first thing you do with it,
is to pay yourself first.
By setting aside a tenth of it.

End of preview.

Preview book Moneymaker

<u>Moneymaker 3</u>

The bible for entrepreneurs, written by an entrepreneur.
So your daily reading.

No, it's not about GOD.

It says, written by an entrepreneur .....

YOU READ ONLY BOOKS WHICH ARE WRITTEN BY PEOPLE WHO HAVE THEIR OWN
COMPANY !!
Do you understand ?

This way you prevent feeding your mind with BULLSHIT.
And that you will model BULLSHIT.
By B.S. I mean unproven idea's and theory.
So you save yourself time and money.

Ok, then a bit about that Entrepreneurial Bible.
It is called No Excuses, the Power of self discipline
And is written by Brian Tracy

And yes, he has his own company.
Otherwise his name would not be here.

It comes down to self discipline.
And self discipline makes you feel very good about yourself.

When you exercise, for example, while most people watch TV.
When you work on a Saturday, while most people have a weekend.
When you take a step towards achieving your goals on Sunday.

The above 3 examples require discipline from you.

But 1, 3, 5 years from now

where will you wind up ?

And where will most people wind up ?

Have you ever worked a day with pain because your teeth were broken?
Have you ever worked with only 2 hours of sleep, the night before?
Have you ever worked without having slept the night before?

It was probably easier to watch TV then .....

But if I did, then I would be a Bullshitter for you,
and not someone who you respect.

I disciplined my self and went to work.

Oh yeah, buy the entrepreneurial bible. NOW.

Previeuw book Moneymaker

<u>Moneymaker 2.</u>

Two things that you have to spend your time on daily

Which 2 are they?

Watch TV and be on Facebook?

Without B.S., so:

SALES & DIRECT MARKETING

If you sell something (sales), then profit comes in.

If you become good at (direct marketing), then profit comes in.

With marketing you save yourself time while selling.
You do not have to explain who you are and what your company does during your presentation.

How many hours per working day do you spend on sales?

How many hours per working day do You spend on Direct Marketing?

WHAT HAPPENS IF YOU ONLY SPEND YOUR WORKINGTIME ON SALES & DIRECT
MARKETING ??

Will you have more profits and therefore more money?

End of preview
For more information about this book by me, go to my website : www.hajrobv.nl

<u>Small introduction with establishment Hajro</u>

Establishment Hajro is committed to helping
the people in the province of Gelderland,
by providing jobs and keeping people working,
by donating to Charities,
and by helping people to live richer.

Today Hajro is
a subsidiary of Hajro Group.

The Hajro Group consists of 20 different companies,
who are all part of
1 umbrella organization.

We now have several products & services,
and we support more than 40 charities.

Visit us at www.hajrobv.nl

and discover what else we can do for you.

Hopefully you will become a raving fan & customer of us.

However you choose,

I wish you

a lot of prosperity & happiness.

Kind regards,

Jasmin Hajro

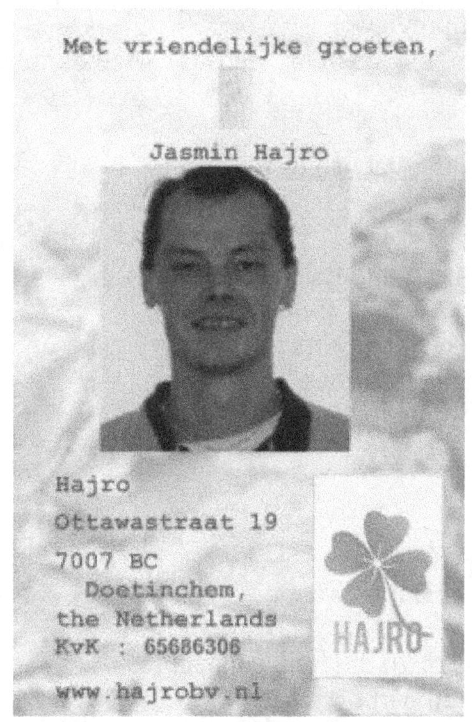

P.S. If you want to let me know your experience
with my book. Send me a message by email to
j.hajro@hotmail.com. Thanx

<u>Overcoming tough times.</u>

<u>The bio of author Jasmin Hajro, nice to meet you</u>

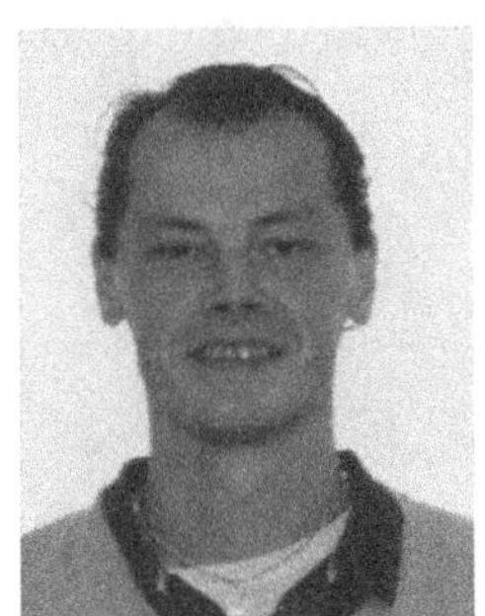

Hello dear reader, how are you ?
Thank you for buying my book.

.

My name is Jasmin Hajro,
I was born on July 6, 1985 in Bosnia.
As refugees, we came to the Netherlands 21 years ago.
After having completed school & worked at several jobs ...

On 17 December 2012, I founded my first company:
investment firm Jasko.
ter a successful first year, I unfortunately had to close that company. After a short period of rest,
unemployment and temporary work. I started again as an entrepreneur.

On September 1, 2015, I founded establishment Hajro.

(We say establishment instead of company,
because we do a bit more than just sell stuff.
Like providing jobs,
donating to 40 different charities,
and helping people to live richer.)

Since the beginning the core activity is,
selling sets of greeting cards, door to door.
Nowadays the product range has been expanded.

With, among other things, the selling of my 12 books.

The royalties of my books are donated to the charity:
foundation Giveth Life.
From there more than 40 other charities receive donations.
And by buying this book you support more than 40 charities.
Thank you.

My company is now part of Hajro Group,
which consists of 19 different subsidiaries,
that are part of 1 umbrella organization :
Called Energy Now. (Energie Nu)

For more information about my company
& the foundation,
go to my website : **www.hajrobv.nl**

<u>Overcoming tough times</u>

What are tough times?

Isn't that different for everyone?

Perhaps something like tiring times.

Times that make you tired.

I worked in a tapas restaurant in Arnhem,

called Ramblas.

The food was delicious,

but I waanted to do something else,

then work in the dishes and the kitchen.

I started a home study for Wft basic Advisor,

when I worked in that restaurant.

In the evening at home I heard that my uncle Ibro,

who lives in Bosnia, had died.

Things were finally going the right way.

I finally had work and earned money,

could pay my bills.

And reduce my debts.

Well then thas bad news came.

It was as if all energy went out of me.

I have very happy memories of

my childhood in Bosnia.

My family is part of my happy memories.

Someone once asked me what I was missing?

Because I had almost no contact with my uncle.

Apparently, those things go like that,

contacts & connections fade ....

Especially if you live far away from each other.

What I missed was his humor,

it always feels good and joyous when I was there.

And going to Bosnia on vacation is no longer

the same, because the people you go for

no longer exist.

I have thought about it...
Because I have already written 11 books.
The one you are reading now is the first part of my new series:
Work to shine.

What kind of book would be good for many people?
What kind of book would be helpful to many people?

What should be in it, what would it have to give to readers?

Even if it is only recognition,
periods I went through &
that they are going through.
That they can relate to.
To know that you can get through anything.
No matter how painful it is
and no matter how bad it seems, at the moment.

Or comfort.

Maybe relativation,
to attenuate their troubles and their situation &
see them in the right perspective.
They're just like a threshold on the road,
that you really will get over.

To be honest, I do not want to write this book.
I do not feel like writing it.
I really had to force myself ,
to sit down &
start writing.

It is Sunday for God's sake.
July 1st
A new month started,
it is beautiful sunny weather outside.

I got up before noon, for once.

Yeah, for some miraculous reasons,
I am almost 33 years old and I still struggle
to get up in the morning on time.

So what does this Workaholic do?
On such a nice Sunday?

Starting on a new book series &
writing a book that he actually does not want to write.

Well if you've read my book Victory,
then you know that one time in Bosnia
when I was a little boy
I had to sit nude in front of the house. As a punishment.

Because of those kind of fokking things,
I did not really want to write this book.

Anyway,
I have already started ....

So what's in it for you, to know what kind of
extreme punishment I received?

Well, whatever is bothering you,
no matter what kind of tough time you're going through now.

Ans no matter how difficult it may be for you ...

ı will never have to sit naked in front of your house,
                  as a punishment.

                    You see,
            your situation is not that bad.

        (That is relativizing, that is to say
    relativation or taking the edge off it)

    Perhaps there is a better translation ?

    But you know what I meant, right ?

Let's go back to Uncle Ibro for a moment,
he left behind a wife and two daughters.

I'm just very sorry that I did not do something for him,
when it was still possible.

I live in a country where I have much more possibilities,
then they have in Bosnia.

I would have liked to send him money every month
And have visited them every year,
or a number of times a year.
Sent them gifts and spent more time with them.

I would have liked him to get to know my great company
& to show him my 11 books which are for sale in 190 countries worldwide...
And the good foundation that I founded.

But that is not possible anymore,
Uncle Ibro is deceased ....

People of gold

For me that was Grandpa Vejsil and Grandma Ziba.
They too lived in Bosnia.
Grandma and step grandpa actually.

Maybe because they have more experience with parenting,
then my parents.
Or because I never got a beating from them.

It was always great fun with grandpa and grandma.

<u>A lot thanks to her</u>

My father's oldest sister, Aunt Rahima.

Thanks to her, we were able to go to the Netherlands.

To get away from the war.

I owe a lot to her.

<u>In a short period of time</u>

In the period of time, that Uncle Ibro died,
I went to work
& then back home again.

I had enough of it
and I left.

In that period,
that lasted perhaps a half year or 1 year.

Aunt Rahima died of cancer,
Grandma Ziba died.

I went to Bosnia and there
I have carried her coffin for a while.

There was a long line of people and the coffin was passed on.
All the way to the grave.

We had a friend of my mother
in our neighborhood: called Ria.

She drank a little too much and had
a strange fear : she was afraid to walk up the stairs.

It was nice with her, when she came to visit.

She also died of cancer.

In that short period of time.

And then I heard that Grandpa Vejsil
also had died.

A while before, grandmother and grandmother had already split up.

But still.

That was 5 people in a short period of time.

At that time we received many letters from collection agencies
and bailiffs.
Our bills that they doubled the amounts that we had to pay
and that was all according to the law.

Yah Yah.

They are legitimate thieves.

So I was very angry and sad then.

Very very angry. Warlike angry.

And sad.

As you understand,
I would have liked to have done something more for them.
Spent more time with them.
Have given them more.

And I would loved to show them,
how far I have come.

From being 1 night homeless,
to writing 11 books & publishing them in 190 countries worldwide
Plus a good foundation &
a company with 16 subsidiaries.

But now it's too late for that.
They are dead.

I stopped using drugs,
after I had taken too much,
and ended up in a coma.

Well if you use yourself or know someone who does that ..
And if you see it as a waste of potential &
want to be clean
or help someone else to become it.

Then it might be good to know,
what I did afterwards.

That was just as important.

I decided, of course, not to do it anymore.
I could not do it anymore.
I think I got an anxiety attack,
when I tried to smoke a blunt.
Because I was shaking,
and wondered if I was going to get a heart attack.

What I did after ...

No more buying that stuff.
Stopped dealing with people who use it.
Yes, I was at home a lot and it was shitty,
but it was better.

I started to become more fanatic with my chess hobby
and kept myself busy with it.

I went for walks.

I thought of people who used as LOSERS

I once collapsed and fell to the ground,
and after that I stopped drinking
alcohol.

What I did after ...
Was not going to the pub anymore.
Didn't go out to clubs anymore.
Drank a lot of tea and coffee.

Went hiking.
I read.
Listened to audiobooks and watched motivational videos
on youtube.

I wrote.

I didn't go anymore to places and people
where alcohol was consumed.

Yes I was a lot of times at home, like a hermit.

But it was better.

Bills and debts

See bills and debts not like a burden,
but as responsibilities.

And people who still have to receive money from you,
are people who trusted you
or have faith in you.

And for that kind of people you are going to make things right.
No matter how much time it takes you.

Put all your bills in 1 folder and put that thing out of sight,
in a drawer or something.

Emplane some cash money around you in your house.

And focus on earning money,
stash money,
and take care of your responsibilities.

<u>Aging sucks</u>

It sucks, right?

Every year, you become a year older.

I thought so too.
And I especially disliked to become 30 years old.
Because I had heard or thought
that after your thirtieth year
you start to decline.
That everything is going to decay and won't function well.

And I thought about, when I become 80 years old,
and nothing functions anymore
to kill myself one way or another.

Until someone said:
The older you get the better it is

And that is the mighty fokking truth,
as far as aging is concerned.

Some children do not even become 10 years old.

Some people don't even become 18 years old.

But you are 30 or 40 or 50 years and having another birthday
& you can live for another year.

How a great gift is that ...
You can do and experience so much. And enjoy.
Be happy
The older you get, the better it is.

<u>The Better thing</u>

Failing and falling on your face is good for you.
And also is rejection.

Because then the Better thing comes on your path.

I had a solution for the banks,
neatly typed out and ready.
They did not want it.

A while after that,
out of my solution I made a book.
book the Lifebuoy for banks
" loyal banking "
(de Reddingsboei voor banken"loyaal bankieren")
The Better thing

I applied for a social wellfare for the 2nd time.
It was rejected.

I walked home,
and then wrote my 3rd book:
book Recipe for Happiness
the Better thing

That is how it will work out for you too.
Do not despair. Work towards your goals and dreams.
The Better thing is coming

<u>a Doing book</u>

Well, as you might already know in the meantime
I write short books.

And Non fiction.
Simply facts and life experiences.

With often things in them that you can do,
or must do.
Actions you can perform,
so that you get results.

You probably already understand that by just
thinking about 10 euros/dollars,
the 10 dollar will not manifest in your pocket.

But if you do something.
Like working for a while.
Then you will receive the 10 dollar.

I would love to recommend to you
my book Recipe for Happiness
(Also a Doing book)

It contains tips and advice that you can easily do &
that help you to have less stress.
To be happier and healthier.

And also help you a bit to overcome difficult times.

<u>Count on one hand</u>

That night on the street is actually the best thing
that has happened to me.

It has put pepper in my ass,
to go to work hard.
And to get more out of myself.

It has also taught me,
that very few people are always there for you.
You can count them on one hand.

Whatever you did,
and however you have behaved.
They are still there for you.

These rare few could be your mom and dad.

Thank them,
appreciate them.

Make some sunshine for them &

make them proud.

Well you now also know with which people you should
spend your time. And not with others.

<u>And that</u>

What I did after I stopped taking drugs and drinking alcohol
was also ...
Working

They were not always the nicest jobs.

But work has really changed my life.

That it will do for you too.

Work is your best friend,
you can always count on it.
You can always 'borrow' money from that friend
after you have worked.

Quote :" Work is the best therapy."
By Doctor Maxwell Maltz

So if you don't believe me, believe the doctor.

<u>Those meager months</u>

And what about those months when you only

earned a few bucks?

I will become a millionaire or die working towards it.

So about really fokking great.

My Victorious series of 10 books &
Another one,
show you:

That if you really want something,
then you can do it too.

No matter what & Whatever they say.

<u>That obvious recipe</u>

It goes something like this:

Write down what you want to achieve in life

Learn, Work & Persist until you realize it

About the same process as getting your driver's license.
Or cooking a meal.
Or getting your diploma.
Or writing a booklet.

Save a part of your money &
donate something to charities.

Keep reading, listening to audiobooks
and developing yourself. Keep growing.

Learn the 80/20 principle,
so that you will only do the most important things,
that give you the most results.

Then you will feel better about yourself &
that also helps you
get thru tough times.

<u>Learn that it does not matter what people say</u>

To achieve the things you want in your life,
the only thing that matters is : what you think and what you DO

If you experience this as a valuable book,
would you please be so kind
to recommend it
to the people that you know.

So that it helps them too with overcoming tough times.

Thank you.

To be the first to know when I bring out a new book,
sign up at the ink below
and you'll get an automatic email
of the grand news…

by Jasmin Hajro (books2read.com)

Sorry if my books are a bit short…
I have given you my best
and poured out my heart and soul
and wrote down my experiences
in life and business…
I hope it all helps you…

I wish for you the best of life.

Kind regards,

Jasmin Hajro

You have read my lifestory….

ıve been fatter because I drunk a lot of beer and ate a lot of food that was fried,
like daily I ate fried french fries….
And I have also been thinner, bacause of excersize and eating more healthy

and now we come to the diet….

I am not a doctor , this advice is just common sense….

‘’It takes 20 minutes of jogging (running) to loose the calories
from eating 1 cookie ‘’

Are you gonna run 20 minutes for every cookie that you eat ?

If you ain’t,
get rid of all the cookies in your house.

Have you got rid of all the cookies ?

In the first month of the diet,
eat only fruit, vegetables and fish

Drink a lot of water….

In the second month eat healthy meals
along with fruit, vegetables and fish

and keep drinking a lot of water.

but like Brian Tracy says :

''get rid of the 3 white poisons in your food''
don't consume any sugar, salt and white flower''

Brian Tracy also says :

''eat less and excersize more''

Join a gym or get a personal trainer
also start taking long walks in your neigbourhood
untill you can start joggin those distances….
Take a walk everyday.

Also take foodsupplements :
multivitams or vitamine A-Z
and minerals…

That you can buy at a drugstore or pharmacy

Take them pills everyday

Get a blender and fruit,
and reward yourself for making the effort
and making progress
by making for yourself a
delicious
smoothie

reward yourself often

Avoid juices that are full of sugar and calories,
drink more water
and coconutjuice
and aloe vera juice

Keep up this new lifestyle for many years !

I hope you liked my booklet
and I really hope that you do the steps
that I suggest,
so that it becomes lifechanging
and your health improves and you lose weight.

Because your health is the most important thing for you.

If you liked my book,
please give some stars as rating
and write something nice about it…
Thank you

More books by Jasmin Hajro :

My bibliography....the books that I have written....

ere are more than 43 titles plus the translations plus the boxsets, so I will only name my english
s)

ld Your Fortune

neymaker

ipe For Happiness

Lifebuoy For Banks "Loyal Banking"

Ultimate Winning Strategy, for entrepreneurs

ich is for salespeople & businessowners too)

ems, jokes and book

tory 1

tory 2

vays employment & always money in your pocket, everyday.

ngs You Don't Want To Know.

allenges in having your own business, in real life.

v to Grow your money & Build a good retirement in 2 hours per month, for moms, dads, career
men and busy people .

ercoming tough times.

crets of writing and selling books.

uble your profits.

uble your profits, extended.

umph 1 (boxset)

umph 2 (boxset)

ctorious series (boxset)

rough the crisis

I don't feel like writing, says the author

Hackers are scouts

Being real and true: in times of fake and pretend

100 % sales rule

Quotes for success

Entrepreneurship course

3

(If you click on them a new window will open, at Lulu, where you learn more about the book

and where you can buy it as paperback or ebook.

If the link doesn't work click here

All my titles are there, but you can search the one that you want..

" I have good experiences ordering at Lulu")

Only available at Amazon and free with Kindle Unlimited are my books :

Lifechanging quotes

the Jasmin Hajro lifestory(which includes Victory 1,2,3,4)

Controversial

This is how you get rich: passively

200 % sales rule

Visit my author website and get 10 free books at

www.jasminhajro6.webnode.nl

Note :

Over the years a few websites have changed….

My author website is now and will always be at

www.jasminhajro6.webnode.nl

You get 10 free books if you visit me there..

My companys website (in dutch) is

www.hajro.be

My companys International website (in english) is :

www.hajro-international.webnode.nl

You are welcome to visit,

maybe there is another great book

or great service for yourselfwaiting there.

Thank you for choosing one of my books to read.

Hopefully you are willing to rate it 4 or 5 stars and give it a positive review.

Thank you so much

for your effort.

I will continue to sell greetingcards

and write more books

untill retirement,

so more good stuff will be available

at my Author website,

www.jasminhajro6.webnode.nl

make sure that you visit it

every year or

more often than that.

Kind regards,

Jasmin Hajro

P.S. I hope this book helps you to change your life..